D0851484

TREAT HER LIKE

a Princess

How to Help Your Girlfriend with Breast Cancer

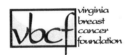

**Gift of the Virginia Breast
Cancer Foundation
2012**

Educate · Advocate · Eradicate

www.vbcf.org
804-285-1200 or 1-800-345-8223

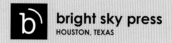

bright sky press
HOUSTON, TEXAS

2365 Rice Boulevard, Suite 202
Houston, Texas 77005

Copyright © 2009 by Denise Hazen. No part of this book may be reproduced in any form or by any electronic
or mechanical means, including information storage and retrieval devices or systems, without prior
written permission from the publisher, except that brief passages may be quoted for review.

10 9 8 7 6 5 4 3 2 1
Library of Congress Cataloging-in-Publication Data
Hazen, Denise, 1964-
Treat her like a princess : how to help your girlfriend with breast cancer / Denise Hazen ;
illustrated by Jennifer Procell ; foreword by Edgardo Rivera.
p. cm.
Includes bibliographical references.
ISBN 978-1-933979-46-5
1. Breast--Cancer--Patients--Care. 2. Caregivers--Popular works. I. Title.

RC280.B8H399 2009
362.196'99449--dc22   2009014908

Edited by Ellen S. Morris and Nora Shire
Designed by Cregan Design
Printed in China through Asia Pacific Offset

TREAT HER LIKE
a Princess

How to Help Your Girlfriend with Breast Cancer

Denise Hazen
Illustrated by Jennifer Procell

Foreword by Edgardo Rivera, M.D.
Chief, Breast Medical Oncology
The Methodist Hospital

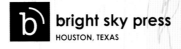
bright sky press
HOUSTON, TEXAS

This book is dedicated to my Knight in Shining Armor, Charles,
and our children, Catherine and Nicholas.

All my love, and always remember:
Every day is a journey, and the journey itself is home.

—Matsuo Basho
(master haiku poet, 1644–1694)

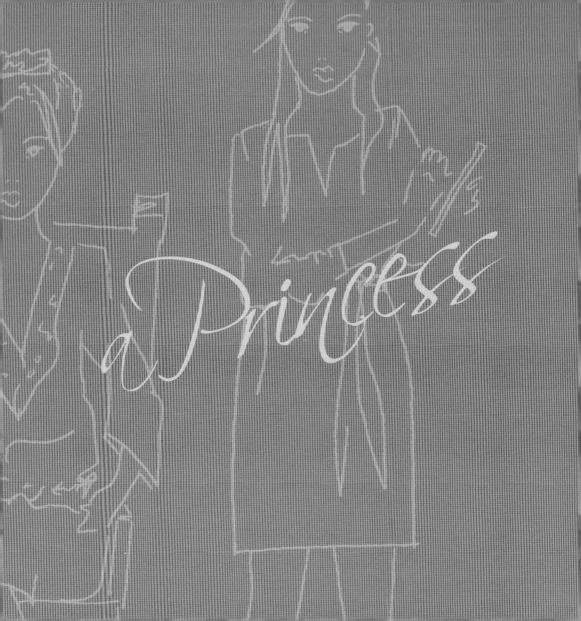

a Princess

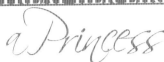
TABLE OF CONTENTS

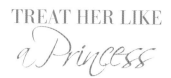
TREAT HER LIKE
a Princess

FOREWORD

It was an honor to be asked to write a foreword for Denise Hazen's book, *Treat Her Like a Princess: How to Help Your Girlfriend with Breast Cancer*. Her personal experience and her keen insight offer a fresh and unique perspective on breast cancer care and compassion and assistance for families and friends of women fighting the disease. Denise brings this perspective to a very complex and challenging facet of the fight for surviving breast cancer. Unlike many of the authors on the subject of breast cancer, Denise successfully reaches out to and educates the cancer patient's support structure and apparatus, ensuring they are made aware of the importance of their role in their "girlfriend's" fight with cancer.

Denise offers wise guidance from the perspective of one who has lived through the experience. For women fighting cancer, she provides a witty mixture of concrete advice and subtle insights about attitude and feeling. It's as though a ballet instructor could instruct you on movement and stance as well as how to think, feel and imagine yourself so that the practical advice blossoms into a prima ballerina. Denise's advice offers that level of sound guidance.

This book is particularly eloquent and helpful about the universal experience of women's difficulty and struggle during the often toxic treatments for fighting breast cancer. I particularly admire Denise's remarkable humor, wit and wisdom when dealing with the subject. She presents it in a way that leads you to know there *is* hope, and that the patient is not alone. Many other women have traveled this road, and they are often more than willing to accept new members to this very unique sorority with open arms and open hearts. Whether you are a woman with breast cancer, her girlfriends or her neighbor, after reading this book you will be better prepared to ensure the maximum results from treatment and care.

As in life, Denise has a strong presence on the page. She wins your heart, your mind and your confidence that her advice is on target. Her approach is all about real life solutions to problems often beyond our control. Denise grabs your attention, then gains your trust and your admiration as she realistically walks you through the many facets of the fight with breast cancer. Her book is about three specific areas that inevitably intertwine during the diagnosis and treatment of breast cancer: optimizing the mind and environment for the fight, educating the patient and her support structure, and preparing the patient for what she will confront during the care and treatment of the disease and using that information to ensure a successful fight.

One of the most telling aspects of Denise's character and personality is conveyed by what is absent from the book. What is not in the book is an in-depth discussion

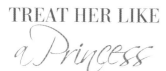
and analysis of *Why Me?* You will not find it in this book, because Denise is not a person who would dwell on or overanalyze why she was diagnosed with breast cancer. Sure, like in life, she spends a brief amount of time dealing with the topic, but she quickly moves on to devoting her full attention and effort to the fight ahead. She knows, and conveys to the reader, that the fight is what is most important after the diagnosis.

I invite you to sit back, open your minds and hearts, and prepare to be educated in a very warm and affirming manner. Let Denise walk with you as you navigate the minefields of breast cancer and prepare you for the fight ahead. You will need all the support you can muster, so use this book to its fullest extent as a resource, as a guide and as advice from a friend. After you walk this journey with Denise through her book, you will most likely see her as a friend and, more importantly, you will know her as a sister in the strong sorority of fighters and survivors of breast cancer.

Edgardo Rivera, M.D.
Chief
Breast Medical Oncology Section
The Methodist Hospital

PROLOGUE

If you are reading this book, either you or one of your girlfriends has been initiated into the sorority that no one wants to join — Crappa Crappa Cancer. Once the "C" word is out there, you might find yourself overwhelmed. What do you do first? Go ahead and get the crying out of your system. You deserve a good cry. Then put the tissues away and get going! You have your work cut out for you, either as the patient or as the support system. *Treat Her Like a Princess* outlines in simple terms how to help the patient and her loved ones deal with the realities of breast cancer as they maneuver through life's daily demands. This guide is intended not only for women facing this challenge, but especially for the women who will stand behind them and lift them up... The Girlfriends.

TREAT HER LIKE
a Princess

Chapter 1
WHY ME?

How could I have breast cancer? For one thing, it wasn't on my agenda. I was too busy to have cancer. And wasn't I too young? Too fit? Too fashionable? My friends would ask me, "why me?" What I learned is that cancer has no prejudice or bias. It affects the young and old, the rich and poor, the fashionistas and glamour don'ts. The American Cancer Society claims that 1 in 3 women have a lifetime probability of developing a cancer and 1 in 8 will develop breast cancer. Why did I think I was exempt? Isn't it funny how we never think it is going to happen to us? To say I was shocked when I was diagnosed with breast cancer is like saying Oscar de la Renta is a tailor. I was quickly thrown into a new world. I felt as if I had traveled to a new country without a travel dictionary. The doctors and nurses started throwing terms at me that even as a Greek woman I couldn't understand. Stage 3—heck, I didn't even know what that meant. Stage 3 out of what? 10? 20? Sentinel node? Hormone receptive?

I realized I had work to do, and with the help of
my family and friends, I strapped on my Jimmy
Choo's and embarked on a journey that I would
have never freely chosen, but one that has
changed me forever, and hopefully for the better.

Through this book, I want to share with
you not only the *how to's* of breast
cancer but also the *how to's* for celebrating
friendships and life.

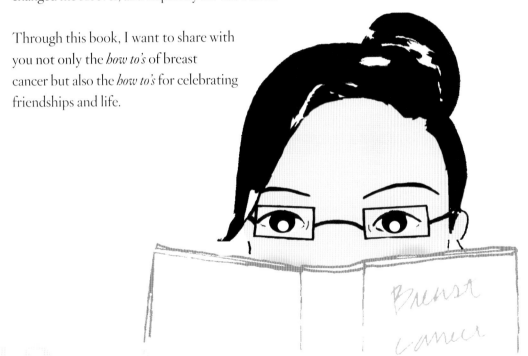

Chapter 2
GETTING ORGANIZED

Believe me, I have always treasured my girlfriends. However, it was not until I was diagnosed with cancer that I found out just how unique the female species is. Within one hour of my diagnosis, phones were ringing off the hook, carpools were being arranged, and food banks set up. My girlfriends were doing what women do best—they were taking charge.

So what do you do when you hear that one of your girlfriends is diagnosed with breast cancer? First and foremost, you let her know that you are willing to help in any way. Then you start making plans.

What does The Princess Need?

Depending on the woman (who will hence be referred to as The Princess) and her situation, the help she will need will differ. Get together with the other girlfriends and decide who will be in charge of which area. That way all calls concerning The Princess will be directed to the right person. The Princess is not in any position to delegate. You must take charge. The "call me when you need me" are nice words, but what she needs right now is **action**.

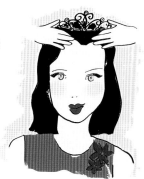

FOOD

Regardless if the woman is single or married, with or without children, she will need to eat. Think about setting up a grocery delivery service and a dinner schedule. This is where consulting with The Princess is important. Find out if she or her family members have any dietary issues. Does she have any cravings, allergies or aversions? Remember this may change throughout her treatment, so check with The Princess periodically.

Bring all food in disposable containers.

15

TREAT HER LIKE
a Princess

RECIPES

Chicken Tortilla Soup — *My girlfriend, Carrie, made this for me during my treatment and it was a hit with the whole family, including me! This is one that I make over and over again for my Princesses.*

- 1   onion, chopped
- 1   jalapeno pepper, chopped
- 2   cloves garlic, minced
- 1   can (14 ½ oz.) stewed tomatoes or tomato sauce
- 4   cups stock (chicken or beef)
- 1   can tomato soup
- 1   teaspoon cumin
- 1   teaspoon chili powder (or less to taste)
-     salt and pepper
- ½   teaspoon lemon pepper
- 2   teaspoons Worcestershire sauce
- 4   corn tortillas, sautéed lightly
- 1   avocado
- 1   can (15 oz.) corn, drained and washed

1   can (15 oz.) black beans, drained and washed
1   rotisserie chicken, cooked & cut into cubes
    Cheddar or Monterey Jack cheese, grated (optional)
    sour cream (optional)

Sauté onion, jalapeno pepper, garlic and tomatoes in a large pot for several minutes. Add remaining ingredients except tortillas, avocado, cheese and sour cream. Simmer for one hour. About 10 minutes before serving, tear tortillas into bite size pieces and add to soup. Place cubed avocado and grated cheese in individual bowls and ladle soup on top. Finish with a spoonful of sour cream.

*This recipe freezes well!

Chicken Pot Pie *— This is great "comfort food" from my girlfriend, Sally!*

8   chicken breasts, bone in & skin on (easier/quicker way, buy rotisserie chicken)
4   tablespoons butter
3   tablespoons olive oil (may need more)
2   med. onions chopped
5   celery stalks
2–3   cups carrots (I use small baby/snack carrots already peeled) sliced thin

TREAT HER LIKE
a Princess

$\frac{1}{4}$ teaspoon fennel seed (I cut seed with knife into smaller pieces)

5 teaspoons "Better Than Bullion"

3-4 tablespoons flour

5 cups milk (whole or skim)

Pillsbury Pie Crust (2) or Puff Pastry from Pepperidge Farm

Place chicken breasts on a sheet pan and rub skin with olive oil. Sprinkle liberally with kosher salt and freshly ground pepper. Roast for 35-45 minutes, until the chicken is just cooked. Set aside until cool enough to handle. Remove meat from the bones, discard the skin and shred into bite size pieces. Set aside.

Saute the onion, celery, carrots and fennel seeds in olive oil and butter. Once translucent, add Better Than Bullion and flour. This should make a paste. Gradually add milk. Let cook med to low heat for approximately 20 minutes. Check consistency; may need more milk or add more flour to thicken. Other vegetables may be added—corn, green beans, potatoes. I like just carrots, onions and celery.

Line round baking dish (approx. 5 in x 12 in) with crust, add chicken mixture, place second crust on top. Seal crust to the edge of baking dish. Cook at 350 for 45–50 minutes.

18

Tortellini Salad—*A great recipe from sister, Vicki, to keep for post surgery visits to the house.*

2–12 oz. packets of tortellini
- 1   8 oz. can or jar of artichoke hearts, drained and cut in $^1/_4$ths
- 1   cup feta cheese

optional:
- $^1/_2$ cup chopped black olives
- $^1/_2$ cup chopped tomatoes

Dressing:
- $^1/_4$ cup white wine vinegar
- $^1/_4$ cup chopped green onions
- 3   medium garlic cloves, minced
- 1   tablespoon dry basil
- 1   teaspoon dry dill
- $^1/_2$ cup olive oil

Cook tortellini according to instructions. Drain. Mix dressing ingredients together. Toss tortellini, artichoke hearts, and feta with dressing. Refrigerate. Tastes really yummy once it has had a chance to marinate in dressing!

19

Chicken Noodle Soup — *another favorite from Sally!*

- 5 tablespoons olive oil
- 1 large onion, chopped
- 5 celery stalks, chopped
- 3 cloves of garlic
- 1 small container of fresh mushrooms, sliced
- 1 sprig of fresh rosemary
- 8 cups of chicken broth/Better Than Bullion
- 1 rotisserie chicken
- 1 12 oz. bag of extra broad noodles or box of Acini Di Pepe pasta
  Kosher salt and pepper to taste

Sauté onion, celery, garlic and rosemary sprig in olive oil until onion and celery are translucent. Add sliced mushrooms (may need to add a little water). Sauté 5–10 minutes. Add chicken broth. Remove meat from rotisserie chicken and add to soup. Bring to boil, then simmer for 10-15; Add noodles/pasta. Serve once noodles/pasta are tender.

Cucumber Soup — *Courtesy of The Soup Lady, Carla!*

3	medium cucumbers, peeled seeded, and cut into chunks
1 1/2	cups chicken broth
1	cup sour cream (use half lite version, half regular)
1/2	cup buttermilk
1/2	cup yogurt
2 1/2	tablespoons white vinegar
1	garlic clove, minced
2	green onions, sliced thin
	salt to taste
2	tablespoons dill, chopped

Process cucumber chunks in food processor with 1/2 cup of chicken broth. Do not over-blend. In a large bowl, combine all remaining ingredients, including the cucumbers. Mix well and chill thoroughly. Makes 5 cups.

*You can add toasted slivered almonds, shrimp or chopped tomatoes too.

TREAT HER LIKE
a Princess

GROCERIES

If a grocery delivery service is available in The Princess'
kingdom, it is a great help. She can log on to the internet
and order what she needs and with the click of a mouse,
her groceries are delivered to her castle. If such a
service is not available in her area, set up your own
version of it. Have The Princess call or email you a grocery list
and then have the girlfriends take turns doing the shopping for her. Make sure to
deliver it and help put it away. Even though The Princess may be able to go to the
grocery on her own, if she is going through chemotherapy, she has no business being
there. It is a germ haven.***

It is also helpful to set up a Target shopping run. Although it is hard to imagine 24
weeks of not seeing the latest fashions from Massimo and Isaac, it's not worth it
for her to be exposed to all that humanity just to buy toilet paper and detergent.
If The Princess has internet access, introduce her to the joys of online shopping.
Encourage her to dream big! Plan ahead for that well-deserved spa vacation, order
birthday gifts or just search for a fabulous new pair of shoes!

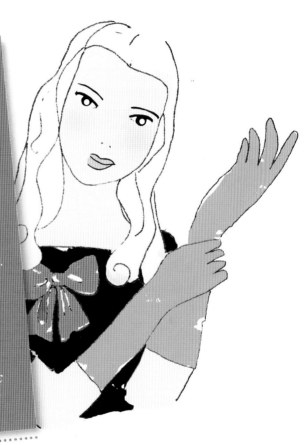

***

Germ Warfare

The Princess must wash her hands often and frequently (this also applies to her subjects).

The Princess must carry an unscented hand sanitizer at all times.

The Princess must bring her own pens with her wherever she goes (who knows what germs lurk at the check out counters).

The Princess needs to don her "white gloves" (or whatever color she desires) when going out to public places.

The Princess does not have to go into hiding but remind her to avoid public places, especially when her counts are low or a flu epidemic is rampant.

TREAT HER LIKE
a Princess

Meals
HOW TO AVOID 50 VERSIONS OF
CHICKEN CASSEROLE

Before you organize her meals, ask The Princess to create a
dining diary, which includes favorite meals (along with recipes if possible), favorite
restaurants and, most importantly, flavors to be avoided!

If you're computer savvy, set up a community calendar on the internet.
Check out www.lotsofhelpinghands.com or www.carecalendar.org.
These services ensure that The Princess' dining needs are met in a
timely and varied manner.

Contact The Princess and see what it is that she will need. Does
she want someone to do the cooking for her? Does her favorite
neighborhood restaurant deliver? Depending on her treatment, she may
have issues with smell, taste, and nausea. ***

Find out her favorite recipes and have a girlfriend post them to the online calendar.
(If the girlfriends are not online, have copies of the recipes available to hand out.)

When someone calls offering to help, they will have the opportunity to donate to the grocery account or to help with the meals. Make sure girlfriends check to see what else has been served that week so all the food groups are well represented. The girlfriends in charge should call The Princess once a week to see what it is that she will need, and they should plan accordingly. Some weeks, she may crave comfort food and home-cooked meals. Other weeks she may be desperate for Moo Shu Pork or Spanakopita. Girlfriends can then take turns picking up food from her favorite haunts.

A practical and efficient tip for the gourmet girlfriends is to make double recipes of their family meal and deliver the other half to The Princess. Soup is a great meal to share because The Princess can freeze it and then pull it out as needed. You will find that sometimes what the family wants to eat isn't what sounds appealing to The Princess. This is another good reason to keep the freezer stocked with quick, favorite, single serving meals.

***

Chemotherapy often changes the palate and the nose. What used to be a favorite of The Princess' might send her running for the porcelain throne.

Chemo may also cause mouth sores, so keep The Princess' freezer full of sugar-free popsicles. Make sure she has plenty of water and straws so that she can stay well-hydrated. Think green and buy The Princess a water filtration system (like Brita) to provide her with chemical-free fresh water while saving the environment. She will need to keep a carafe by her bed too!

Chapter 3
FOLICALLY CHALLENGED

When The Princess is first diagnosed with cancer, she will be faced with many unknowns. However, one thing is certain. If The Princess is undergoing chemotherapy, she is going to lose her hair. The anticipation of losing her Rapunzel-like locks will most likely be stressful for The Princess. It will be a daily reminder of what is going on inside and outside her body. The Princess will need her most glamorous and goodhearted girlfriends to accompany her to the wig shop before she loses her hair. (That way they can try to match the color and cut of her hair.) Before she goes, have The Princess get a prescription from her oncologist for the wig. Most insurance companies will reimburse for one wig.

Wigs have come a long way, Baby! The Princess will find that wigs come in a huge variety of colors and cuts. If she has ever wondered if blondes really do have more fun, now might be the time for her to find out! This may also be the perfect opportunity to try out the latest hair trends! The Princess may want to be daring

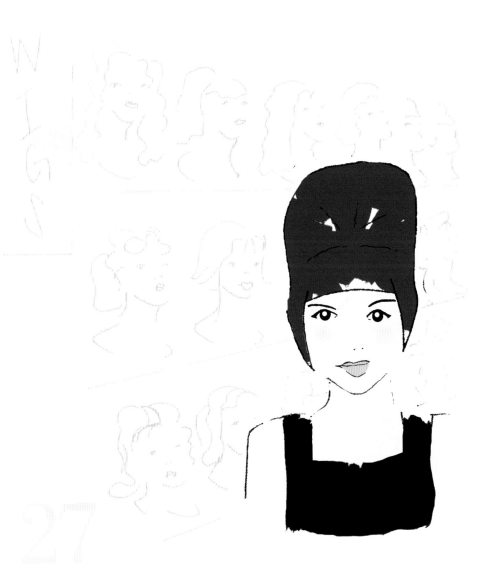

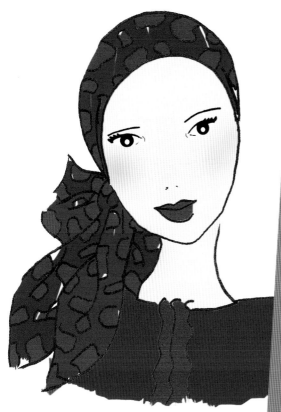

Wearing (or not wearing) a wig is a personal decision. Please be respectful of The Princess' choice and support her. You can help her by making sure she is well-stocked with becoming hats, baseball caps, scarves and durags.

In the event that The Princess must attend a Ball, suggest a black bowler-type hat or a beautiful silk scarf.

If she chooses to go au natural, big earrings can make her feel more feminine.

***

Don't forget that all of her hair on her body will most likely fall out. Forget about making a bikini wax appointment but do go to the drug store and buy her some fake eyelashes. The inexpensive ones work great. Just be sure not to get the super long ones or The Princess will look like a drag queen!

with her wigs. Encourage her to have fun with it! Ask the salesperson to describe the pros and cons of synthetic versus real hair to help The Princess with her decision. After The Princess has purchased her wig, she will probably want to have it cut and styled to frame her face.

Depending on The Princess' treatment plan, she may lose her hair after her first treatment, or it may thin over several treatments. Most patients opt to have their head shaved once the majority of their hair has fallen out. One thing The Princess will notice once she starts chemotherapy is that her hair will actually "hurt." This is usually the signal for hair loss. Because hair tends to fall out evenly, remind her to brush her hair. The Princess may be reluctant for fear of speeding up the hair loss process. However, brushing will help to keep the hair from matting.

*Once The Princess has lost her hair, she can buy Nioxin Scalp Recovery serum to put on her head when she showers. This has been shown to stimulate hair growth. Once her hair begins to grow back, buy her shampoo with nioxin in it. Many beauty supply stores carry this.

TREAT HER LIKE
a Princess

****An organic hair tonic recipe for dry skin:*

1. Wash head with baby shampoo only.
2. Prepare a mixture of $\frac{1}{2}$ antiseptic (like Seabreeze) and $\frac{1}{2}$ bottled water. Pat the mixture onto the head gently with a wash cloth.
3. Apply ISOPLUS Castor Oil Hair & Scalp Treatment (available at beauty supply stores and some grocery stores) to head. Using fingertips, massage well, working upward from the nape of the neck to the top of the head.

Make sure The Princess doesn't shave her head all the way (*The King and I* style). This will save her from ingrown hairs. If The Princess has this done at a salon, make sure a girlfriend goes with her. Tell The Princess to wear her favorite, most flattering color and have a full face of makeup, including lipstick to the salon. This will be a very emotional time for The Princess, but it may also be a relief. The anticipation of losing one's locks is often worse than the actual loss. After the salon, do not take The Princess home right away. Give her time to absorb the trama of losing her hair. Arrange with the other girlfriends a get together. Have everyone bring her hair accessories, hats, scarves, an assortment of bandanas, or durags.

*When the Princess goes to have her hair shaved, think about printing up some hilarious "bad" hairdos! Ask Princess if she would like to take a "walk on the wild side" and see what she would look like with a mullet or mohawk before the final shave. The few minutes of comic relief might help to make the experience less painful.

*There was a reason why men use to wear nightcaps to bed! Bald heads get cold! Visit *www.planetbuff.com* for headwear for the Princess to slumber in and wear around the house.

POST CHEMOTHERAPY HAIR

The Princess will find that her new locks resemble down feathers more than the hair she has always known. This hair (called chemo hair) is very soft and fuzzy and often comes in very curly. The Princess' hair may not resemble her hair prior to chemo. Hair often grows back different colors and textures. Remind her that the last place for her hair to grow back is around the forehead and bangs area. However, within a year, most hair returns to its prior texture.

TREAT HER LIKE
a Princess

*The Princess may hesitate to have her hair trimmed once it begins to come in. Encourage her to have it shaped to avoid a "Bozo the clown" look.

*In order for her hair and head to accept the change of the new hair growth, she needs to wear her wig less and less. The Princess should surf the internet for fun "short" hair dos. Encourage her to buy hair products to spike her hair! Don't forget about cute barrettes and headbands!

***Remind her, the shorter the hair, the bigger the earrings!!!

HAIR COLORING

The Princess must check with her doctor before having any color or chemicals applied to her hair.

When she is given the ok, she must understand that chemo hair takes color differently from other hair. The Princess will most likely have to wait 3 to 4 months before she is able to have hi lights.

***A great (and safe) product to help The Princess restore her lush lashes is Enormous Lash by Beauty Society. Visit *www.beautysociety.com* for more information on their products.

Chapter 4
SUPER FREAK

One thing we as women do not do well is put ourselves first. The Princess must realize that in order for her to be able to do all that she had once done, she needs to make herself and her health her first priority. This is where the girlfriends' power is really important. The girlfriends must sit The Princess down and tell her how they are going to manage all the other areas for her. The Princess may be reluctant to give over control, but be persistent. Now is not the time to be Super Woman!

Here are some ways you can help:

THANK-YOU NOTES

Personal thank-you notes reflect good training, but remind The Princess that now is not the time to worry about pleasing her mother or Miss Manners.

An easy solution to the thank-you note dilemma is to have notes preprinted with a "thank you for thinking of me during this time" inscription and The Princess' name. A girlfriend can then keep up a list of supporters and well-wishers and address and mail the notes. Every Princess deserves a personal secretary at least once in her life!

*Buy several different gifts that The Princess can keep to give for birthdays or special occasions. Wrap them or put them in gift bags with a sticky note describing what the gift is.

Scheduling
DOCTORS APPOINTMENTS

Make sure someone is always with The Princess for her doctors appointments. If a family member cannot go with her, make other arrangements. Have all questions for the doctor written down prior to the appointment. Whoever takes her will need to take notes on all that the doctor reports. Buy a notebook for The Princess that she can take to all her doctors appointments. Often, doctors will allow you to record the appointments. Ask if that is a possibility. Don't forget to request copies of any lab reports. Any notes taken, lab reports, or questions she has for the doctor can be neatly organized in her notebook and will be easily accessible.

TREAT HER LIKE
a Princess

*Questions to think about asking doctors

1. What type of cancer do I have? Is it hormone sensitive? Her-2 positive?
2. What is the size of my tumor? Has it spread to my lymph nodes?
3. What are my options for treatment?
4. Why have you chosen this treatment?
5. What are the risks involved? Side effects?
6. Do you have any suggestions to ease the side effects?
7. How will the treatment affect my daily life?
8. Are there alternative treatments?
9. Are there any clinical trials I can participate in?
10. What is the time line for my treatment?
11. How can I get ready for treatment?
12. Should I consider family history in choosing my treatment plan?
13. Do you suggest a lumpectomy or mastectomy? What are the benefits and risks?
14. Will the treatment cause early menopause? Infertility?
15. Should I do chemotherapy before or after surgery? Why?
16. Are there any medications or supplements I should avoid during treatment?
17. Can I get a copy of my pathology report?
18. Can I exercise during treatment?
19. What should I avoid during treatment?
20. What is the post-treatment follow up care plan?

36

*Keep tract of all doctors, nurses and clinic numbers. Find out what to do in case of a medical emergency. Know where The Princess is to go if she finds herself in need of immediate attention. Ask the doctors to tell you what they consider an emergency? Fever over 100?

*Chemotherapy often causes insomnia. Ask the doctors to give The Princess a prescription for a sleeping aid. If they do not, ask them what they recommend for The Princess to get her beauty rest?

*Cancer Hospitals offer patient advocates, who act in behalf of the patient. Find out who The Princess' advocate is and keep her number close by. Make sure someone other than The Princess has access to this and call the advocate when questions concerning The Princess' care arise.

*The Princess may decide to have genetic testing depending on her family history, type of cancer or personal reasons. This is a very emotional decision for her. Be supportive and understanding. She can visit *www.facingourrisk.org* for more information and support for women who are genetically at high-risk for breast and ovarian cancer.

37

TREAT HER LIKE
a Princess

*Help The Princess to remember to take her medicine (and keep track of what medicines she has already taken) by providing her with a chart or a labeled pill box.

	Sun–am	Mon–am	Tues–am	Weds–am	Thurs–am	Fri–am	Sat–am
Medication							
1.							
2.							
3.							
4.							
5.							

	Sun–mid day	Mon–mid day	Tues–mid day	Weds–mid day	Thurs–mid day	Fri–mid day	Sat–mid day
Medication							
1.							
2.							
3.							

	Sun–pm	Mon–pm	Tues–pm	Weds–pm	Thurs–pm	Fri–pm	Sat–pm
Medication							
1.							
2.							
3.							

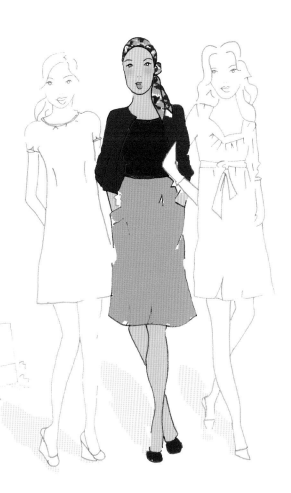

*If you do not live near The Princess, offer to send a car service to drive her to and from appointments when she is unable to drive herself.

CHEMO BUDDIES

You will find this to be one of the girlfriends' favorite duties. It is a chance for you to have several hours of uninterrupted time together with The Princess (with the exception of the nurses). There will be no phones ringing or kids screaming, just a chance to really visit or sit there and chill together. Make sure The Princess knows that you are there to keep her company, not the other way around. If she needs to sleep, let her.

39

TREAT HER LIKE
a Princess

KIDS

If The Princess has children, one of the biggest challenges she will face is how to deal with them without completely turning their lives upside down. Being honest with the children about the changes her body will go through, starting with the loss of hair through the lack of energy, will most likely make cancer seem less frightening. Often the fear of not knowing is worse than the facts. Talk to The Princess and see how she wants to handle this, and respect her decision.

The Year My Mother Was Bald by Ann Speltz is a helpful book for 8-12 year olds. It is written from the perspective of a child whose mother is undergoing

It is important if you are the chemo buddy that you come prepared. Make sure that you bring bottled water, crackers (peanut butter, cheese, Wheat Thins, etc.) and lots of reading material: preferably ones that are just good eye candy-like People, InStyle, US, etc. Also check to see if the hospital or clinic has DVD players in the infusion rooms. There is nothing like a great chick flick to help pass the infusion time. Just make sure to preview for content. Make certain it is uplifting and doesn't have a cancer theme.

***

Before you pick up The Princess for her treatment, encourage her to get gussied up! Her attitude toward treatment will be more positive if she looks like a supermodel!

How to Help Your Girlfriend with Breast Cancer

breast cancer treatment. *Our Mom Has Cancer* by Abigail Ackerman is also good for younger children.

*Find out when major projects, like History or Science Fair, are due and offer to take children to get art supplies and help them complete.

*Check with The Princess' hospital to see if they offer counseling services for children. Often support groups can offer children a chance to express their fears and anxieties, as well as providing them a forum with other children in their position.

LUNCHES

If The Princess' children have a hot lunch program at their school, now would be a great time to enroll them. If they do not, get together with the other girlfriends and find out what the children like to eat and take turns fixing the lunches. For example, PB and J sandwiches can be made in bulk and frozen. All The Princess has to do is pull them out as needed. You can also make single-serving meals like soup and pasta that can be frozen and used as needed.

Girlfriends can also take turns making weeks worth of lunches. All non-perishables can be put in individually labeled bags. Then all The Princess has to do is put each item into lunch boxes each morning.

TREAT HER LIKE
a Princess

CARPOOLING

Find out The Princess' children's schedules and coordinate with one another. If you find that there are some areas that do not have drivers, call your local university or community college and see about posting an advertisement for a college student who could be a driver. A calendar of events and drivers will help keep this organized. If the Princess is unable to drive herself to her children's activities, offer to give her a ride.

HOMEWORK

Homework is a scary endeavor even on our best days! Imagine dealing with it when you are feeling less than stellar. Offer to help The Princess. Depending on the children's ages, suggest forming a study group at school or at someone's home. The children can get their homework finished together and quiz each other for upcoming tests. You will find this to be beneficial for your children as well as The Princess'. Plus, the children will learn how to help others while getting their work completed too!

Check at the child's school to see if there is someone who would be willing to stay after and help. Again, check with the local universities to see if there are any students interested in tutoring.

ACTIVITIES

It is very important for the children to continue with their activities, if possible. Finding drivers may seem like a daunting task, but you will be surprised at how many people are willing to help. Just ask! For example, when the owner of the gym where my children took gymnastics found out that I was undergoing treatment, she offered to take and bring my children home. That was a huge blessing because my children were able to keep doing something that they loved.

CANDY CHEMO COUNTDOWN

Here is a suggestion to help kids understand the length of treatment. Explain how many weeks of chemo or radiation mom will have. Buy them each a jar and fill it with their favorite candy or treat, one piece for every day of mom's treatment. Each day they will be allowed to take one piece of candy or treat. When the jar is empty, mom's treatment is finished!

TREAT HER LIKE
a Princess

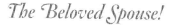

The Beloved Spouse!

Sometimes known as The Forgotten One. Many times, Prince Charming is often overlooked. For most men, it is very difficult to see their Princess suffer. Not being able to "fix it" will be a challenge. We, as girlfriends, have to make sure that they, The Guy Friends, get Prince Charming out of the house. Have the guys take him out for dinner or drinks every few weeks. Organize a golf or tennis match. Find out what Prince Charming's interests are and help coordinate outings. The spouse needs to be able to escape from the world of cancer for a while too. Set up a poker night. Check the local movie theaters. Surely, there has got to be at least one macho film playing!

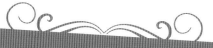

> The Princess and The Prince need time to reconnect outside the doctors' offices and hospitals. If one of the girlfriends has a vacation home, offer it to The Prince and The Princess for an overnight escape. If they have children, hire a babysitter or offer to take the kids for a few hours so they can go out to dinner, if possible, or a movie.

*Often the significant other feels left out and insecure of his role. Be careful not to judge Prince Charming. Remember that he is going through this too.

*An excellent resource for spouses is *Breast Cancer Husband* by Marc Silver. Make a "goodie bag" for Prince Charming and include a copy. He deserves to feel loved too.

PETS

Don't forget Fido or Fifi! If The Princess owns a pet, offer to take it to the vet or groomers. Take turns with other pet-loving girlfriends and make sure the pet is getting exercise.

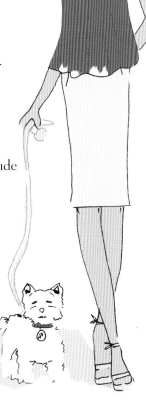

45

TREAT HER LIKE
a Princess

*If you live outside of the Princess' domain, see if there are mobile pet groomers and/or professional dog walkers available.

CASTLE CONTROL

Scrubbing sinks and bathtubs may tarnish The Princess' tiara. If the Princess does not have a house-keeper, get together with the other girlfriends and collect money for a cleaning service. Assess what The Princess' needs are and plan accordingly.

If hiring a cleaning service isn't in your budget, gather a few friends, put on your tiaras and hot pink rubber gloves. Blare some good tunes (think Madonna's "Borderline" or Gloria Gaynor's "I Will Survive") and have a cleaning party. It doesn't seem like work when you are together having fun!

*If The Princess lives alone, supply her with paper plates and plastic utensils. After each meal she can easily dispose of them without the worry of washing dishes.

****Think how surprised Princess will be when she returns from treatment and sees a yard planted with beautifully colored flowers. Surely there is at least one girlfriend with a green thumb who can spruce up Princess' yard! It might be as simple as a new potted plant by the door or a colorful hanging basket. Princess will be able to enjoy the flowers for weeks to come!

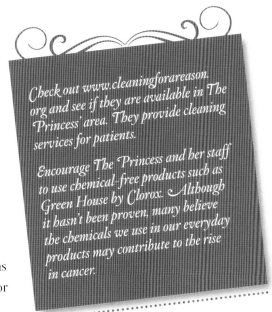

Check out www.cleaningforareason.org and see if they are available in The Princess' area. They provide cleaning services for patients.

Encourage The Princess and her staff to use chemical-free products such as Green House by Clorox. Although it hasn't been proven, many believe the chemicals we use in our everyday products may contribute to the rise in cancer.

Is it holiday season? The Princess will feel better if her castle is festive. Get a group together and deck the halls! How about being a "Secret Santa?" Everyone loves surprises. Drop off treats at her domain with a note attached that says..."on the first day of Christmas..." and continue for twelve days. Hot cocoa mix, supplies to make s'mores, peppermint sticks all make fun gifts! Make sure that no one inside her castle gets a look at "Santa" until the twelfth day! The mystery will drive them crazy!

INSURANCE CLAIMS

Trying to maneuver through the insurance system can cause much strife. If there is a girlfriend who is familiar with dealing with the ins—and outs—of insurance nuances, have her help The Princess.

Set up a medical expense file for The Princess to keep all her receipts and bills. As one of my daughter's beloved teachers would say, "Organization is the key to success in life!"

*Don't be afraid to ask doctors for samples of medication. Call the drug companies and ask for samples or coupons. Check to see if The Princess' insurance company offers mail order prescriptions. Often these services offer medications at discounted prices.

See pages 106–107 for charts to help organize The Princess and her Court.

THE PRINCESS OF WORK

Continuing to work during treatment will be a personal decision for The Princess. She may want to work to try to keep her life as "normal" as before the "C" word. She may not have the financial freedom to take a leave of absence. The side effects of the treatments she is enduring may also play a large role in her ability to work. Find out how you can help her. Does she need help financially? Does she need you to pick up an extra shift so she can have more time off to recover? Does she need someone to help her communicate to her boss the extent of her treatment?

*Provide The Princess' workplace with antibacterial soap and gel. Remember to keep your distance if you are harboring a cold or fighting off the flu.

***If The Princess is single or finding it hard to make ends meet, flowers may not be what she needs. Get together with the other girlfriends and set up an account for her everyday expenses. The Princess may not be able to keep up with the rising costs of medical co-pays, prescriptions and hospital parking. Daily expenses such as rent, utilities and groceries may be difficult to pay, especially if she is unable to work full-time.

49

TREAT HER LIKE
a Princess

Chapter 5

PAMPERING THE PRINCESS

Remember not to pity The Princess or treat her like a sick person. Instead, celebrate your friendship by pampering her.

Think about planning a girlfriend trip or a party to kick off her treatment. Make T-shirts and hats that you can all wear in support of The Princess. Leave off the pink ribbons and come up with logos or slogans that will make her laugh. How about printing up bumper stickers in her support! The Princess is sure to feel loved when she drives about town and sees the stickers.

*Visit *www.thera-wear.com* for awesome T-shirts, napkins and other goodies with inspiring quotes.

*Buy mugs with smiley faces or an image of Super Woman and pass them around the office, gym or carpool line in The Princess' honor. Make your own mug at the

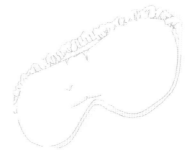

local photo shop with a picture of The Princess and her girlfriends or with an inspiring quote like "embracing my inner princess!"

There are websites that allow you to make your own version of the "Livestrong" bracelets. Have them made in The Princess' favorite color and with her favorite quote.

*Keep all conversations positive and only tell her survivor stories. Now is not the time to tell her about women who have lost the battle. Please—no "Debbie Downer" stories.

*Plan a dinner party and require each guest to wear a shower cap!

*Provide The Princess with Gift Cards so she can go shopping when she needs some retail therapy!

51

TREAT HER LIKE
a Princess

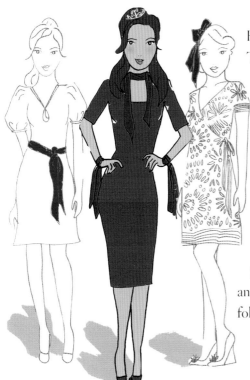

Here a few suggestions for indulging The Princess.

The Scarf Party

Arrange a get-together with The Princess. Prior to the party (without The Princess' knowledge) have each girlfriend pick a favorite scarf to give to The Princess. Each guest is to wear the chosen scarf to the party. (Get creative here, girls! You can tie it in your hair, around your neck or purse!) As the party progresses, have one girlfriend take off her scarf and give it to The Princess. The rest of you can follow suit. Depending on how astute

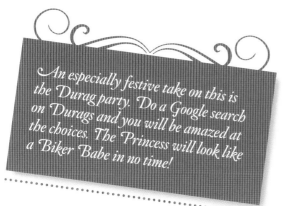

An especially festive take on this is the Durag party. Do a Google search on Durags and you will be amazed at the choices. The Princess will look like a Biker Babe in no time!

The Princess is, it may take her a moment to realize what is happening. Once she understands that her girlfriends have once again put her on a throne, she will be speechless.

(This party can also be done with hats and baseball caps.)

THE DO-IT-YOURSELF PRINCESS KIT

One of the side effects of chemo can be headaches. Make sure The Princess has her Princess Kit (eye mask and ear plugs) prior to chemo. Insist that she retire to her chambers on the days that she is not feeling well. Instruct her to put on her Princess gear, unplug the phones and rest. Remind her that she must nap daily. Sleep is nature's way of healing the body!

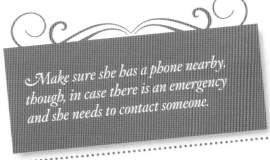

Make sure she has a phone nearby, though, in case there is an emergency and she needs to contact someone.

TREAT HER LIKE
a Princess

ENTERTAINMENT

This will depend on The Princess. She may enjoy a good read or maybe just be up for a lighthearted chick flick. Girlfriends can make movie runs for her; however, there are a few caveats to this. One, make sure you know what kinds of movies she likes to watch (a documentary on the migration of the sperm whales may not be her thing!). Two, read the synopsis. Now is not the time to watch *Stepmom* or *Terms of Endearment.*

Nothing makes you feel better than watching a great chick flick with one or more of your girlfriends. Make a date with The Princess, get comfy, grab a bowl of popcorn and escape from reality for a few hours.

Here is a list worthy of the Chick Flick's Hall of Fame:

For retro fun
"Pillow Talk," "That Touch of Mink," "Lover Come Back," "Sabrina," "Breakfast at Tiffany's" and "Funny Face."

54

For the romantic

"Pride and Prejudice" — the 6-hour special from the BBC is the ultimate! The remake is also great. Check out the Bollywood version called "Bride and Prejudice!" It is hilarious! Another romantic classic is "A Room with a View!"

Movies that make us feel great

"The Princess Bride," "Never Been Kissed," "About a Boy," "When Harry Met Sally," "Under the Tuscan Sun," "13 going on 30," "The Holiday," "Shall We Dance," "My Big Fat Greek Wedding," "While You Were Sleeping," "Pretty Woman," "My Best Friend's Wedding," "The Truth About Cats and Dogs," "Bridget Jones' Diary and French Kiss."

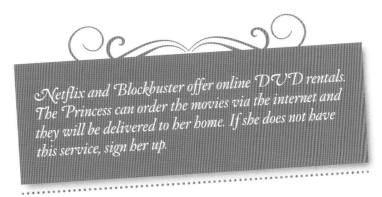

Netflix and Blockbuster offer online DVD rentals. The Princess can order the movies via the internet and they will be delivered to her home. If she does not have this service, sign her up.

55

TREAT HER LIKE
a Princess

LOUNGING IN STYLE

Being the Super Woman that she is, The Princess probably doesn't own proper lounge wear.

Warm-ups and tank tops are comfortable and easy to layer. (One of the side effects of chemo is hot flashes, so she needs to be able to strip quickly when one hits her!) If that is not a staple in her wardrobe, make sure she has a few sets. (Comfy PJ's and non-skid slippers are also a must.)

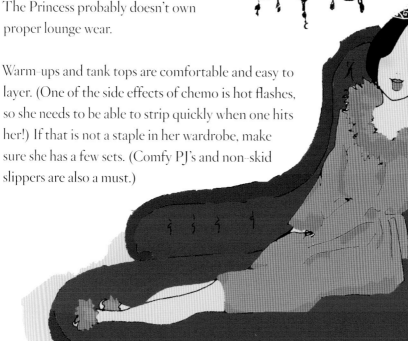

Thinking of Yous

Use your imagination and take into consideration what might brighten up The Princess' day. For those of you who need a little guidance, here are a few suggestions.

CARDS

There are so many great girlfriend-inspired cards. Take the time to find the perfect one for The Princess and send it to her. Just think about how touched she will be when she finds a special card amongst all the junk mail and bills.

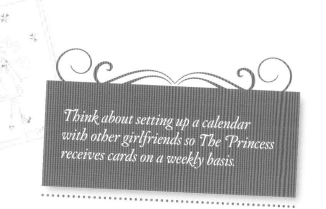

Think about setting up a calendar with other girlfriends so The Princess receives cards on a weekly basis.

GIFTS

They do not need to be extravagant to be meaningful to The Princess. Think about leaving a blooming plant on her doorstep or a dozen freshly baked cookies. Just knowing that someone is thinking about her will brighten up her day. Don't overload The Princess with technical and heavy-duty books on breast cancer. Find uplifting and inspiring books instead.

TREAT HER LIKE
a Princess

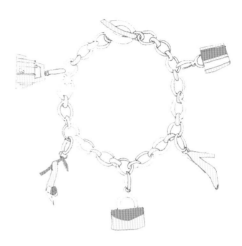

GOOD LUCK CHARMS

Ask the girlfriends to each come up with a good luck charm for The Princess to carry with her to appointments, treatments and hospital stays. Each girlfriend will have her own unique charm. Some may bring a religious token, others an uplifting quote, maybe a stuffed animal or even a favorite photo of loved ones in a beautiful frame. The sky is the limit. Have each girlfriend write a small note explaining why she chose her talisman for The Princess.

Not all Princesses are ready to change their wardrobes to pink. Some Princesses may not want constant reminders of their new sorority. Think twice before making The Princess the poster child for breast cancer.

*During her treatment The Princess is unable to go for manicures and pedicures in salons. Arrange to have someone come to her and pamper her in the comfort of her own castle. The Princess can provide her own tools and polish to avoid any germs.

Now is the time The Princess really needs the royal treatment

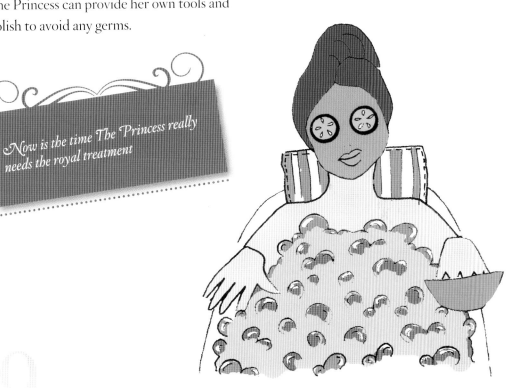

Chapter 6
SPIRITUAL SUPPORT

Think about starting a new tradition by giving The Princess something that she can cherish during her treatment. After she has completed her treatment, she can then pass the item on to someone else facing the same challenges. The Princess can share her treasure as well as her experiences and words of advice and encouragement.

Look for a soft blanket that The Princess can put in her bag to take to appointments and treatments. Having a familiar "lovey" will bring her warmth in more ways than one.

The Princess may find comfort in her spiritual belief system. Some women find comfort through their churches, synogues and mosques. Others find support through meditation, mantras and affirmations. Find out what will help The Princess and respect her choices.

I was given a book by a fellow breast cancer patient who I met during my treatment. I continue to pass the book, *Everyday Strength, A Cancer Patient's Guide to Spiritual Survival* by Randy Becton, along to other's facing the challenges of cancer. The book offers short anecdotes and daily prayers. Another favorite is, *Jesus Calling* by Sarah Young.

*If The Princess has a strong faith and is facing an important doctor's appointment or surgery, think about dropping off a bracelet with a treasured bible verse or a prayer bracelet. It will give her strength and reassurance as she glances down. If she is of a different faith from yours, now is the time to learn about her religious beliefs.

*Maybe there is a symbol, bible verse or mantra that will encourage and empower The Princess. Make sure she has a daily reminder of it.

***The Outreach of Hope ministry offers cancer patients inspirational support materials as well as prayer support. Started by San Francisco Dodger's pitcher, Dave Dravecky, after he lost his pitching arm to cancer, the ministry provides an "Encouragement Basket" to cancer patients free of charge.

TREAT HER LIKE
a Princess

A few of my favorite bible verses that offer hope include:

- "...and lo, I am with you always."
- "I can do all things through Christ who strengthens me."
- "I know every thing about you—even to the numbers of hair on your head."
  (This verse has great significance once The Princess begins to lose her hair.)
- "A cheerful heart is good medicine, but a crushed spirit dries up the bones."

*Consider buying The Princess a "hope chest" or "a sunshine box." Fill it with meaningful and inspiring books, favorite photos, CDs, scripture verses, and prayers. The Princess can open it up all at once or just take things out one at a time as she needs them. Hopefully, the Princess will be reminded of her many blessings on her down days and be thankful for the wonderful gift of friendship.

*Think about making a photo album for The Princess celebrating your friendship through the years and writing why she is special to you. Or maybe just write her a letter letting her know how much you cherish her.

My sister-in-law, Helene, wrote me a beautiful poem called Sea Glass while I was undergoing treatment. I was forever touched by its beauty and significance. Special poems will touch The Princess too.

Sea Glass

Once whole and complete, you
now find yourself shattered and displaced.
Recklessly tossed into the sea,
shards of you are scattered onto the ocean floor,
and what seemed like an end proved only to be a beginning.
The capricious waves take you on a journey—
a long and somewhat tedious ride in which you have
surrendered yourself to the forceful currents.

Pitched about the infrastructure of the sea,
you collide with coral reefs and shells
and pieces of you are chiseled away.
You no longer know where you are or what is left of you
And this journey seems without end.

But then a piece of you finds solitude
in the gentle caresses of the sand.
Your jagged edges are smoothed and your color is purified.
With each ebb and flow of the sea,
Your beauty emerges like a clear, blue sky
after days of torrential rains.

Until one day you find yourself washed up on the shore,
hidden amongst the stones and shells responsible for your fine-tuning.
You are different, yet you are the same.
You are a concentrated version of what you were before.
Yet will you be seen? Really seen?
And so you lay waiting... waiting...
waiting for someone with an eye for raw and pure beauty
to come along and discover you glistening in the sun.

Now you are the envy of all others on the beach—
The sand dollars are broken,
the seashells are only a hint of what they used to be.
But you appear more radiant than ever.
Your journey was not in vain.
You were carried by your Faith through the perils of the sea
and as you rest on the sand,
you appreciate a peace and calm like never before
knowing that you can endure anything
so long as you are willing to be carried...

TREAT HER LIKE *a Princess*

Attitude

There once was a woman, who woke up one morning,
Looked in the mirror,
And noticed she had only three hairs on her head.
"Well," she said, "I think I'll braid my hair today!"
so she did and she had a wonderful day!

The next day she woke up,
Looked in the mirror,
And saw that she had only two hairs on her head.
"Hmm!" she said,
"I think I'll part my hair down the middle today!"
so she did and she had a grand day!

The next day she woke up,
Looked in the mirror,
And noticed that she had only one hair on her head.
"Well," she said,
"today I'm going to wear my hair in a ponytail!"

The next day she woke up,
Looked in the mirror,
And noticed that there wasn't a single hair on her head.
"Yea!" she exclaimed,
"I don't have to fix my hair today"
Attitude is everything!
Be kinder than necessary,
For everyone you meet is fighting some kind of battle.

Live simply,
Love generously,
Care deeply,
Speak kindly...
Leave the rest to God!

Life isn't about waiting for the storm to pass...
It's about learning to dance in the rain!

TREAT HER LIKE
a Princess

*Give Princess permission to mourn. Mourning is a natural part of the treatment process. Princess has lost a lot due to this disease. Her life will forever be changed. Let her know you are there to hold her up during these times. Think about going to her home when she is feeling down and asking her to give you her troubles "to hold" for a while. Tell her to rest and that you will carry the burden for her while she sleeps.

E-MAIL

E-mail is a great, inexpensive way to check up on The Princess' progress and let her know that you are thinking of her. The Princess can check the messages at her leisure. If she is overwhelmed by the amount of e-mail, have a girlfriend print them and put them in a folder for The Princess to view at a later time. Please do not be offended if she does not respond to each and every e-mail she is sent. If at all possible, have a girlfriend in charge of reporting The Princess' progress. One way to do this is to create a personal profile on either Facebook or Carepages. com. The "Webmaster" can update it periodically. This will save The

Princess from having to retell her situation over and over. These sites allow friends and loved ones to check on The Princess as well as to allow them to send words of encouragement and inspiration without requiring a royal reply.

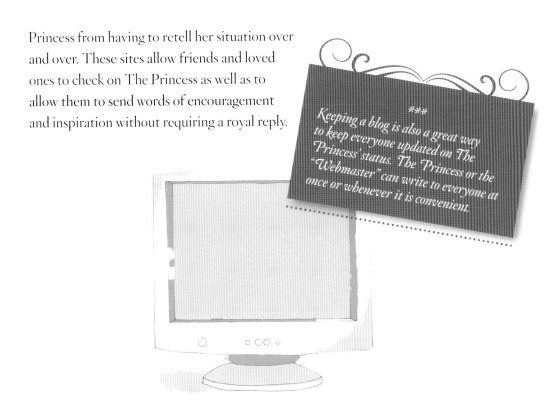

***

Keeping a blog is also a great way to keep everyone updated on The Princess' status. The Princess or the "Webmaster" can write to everyone at once or whenever it is convenient.

Chapter 7
CHEMOTHERAPY SIDE EFFECTS

CHEMO BRAIN

This is a well-documented phenomenon that will most likely cause The Princess much angst. She may find herself struggling for words or having difficulty recalling what she had for breakfast. (I still claim chemo brain on occasion. It beats senility!)

***
Before The Princess begins chemotherapy, have her go to her dentist for a cleaning or any other dental work she may need. Once her treatment begins, she will not be able to have any dental procedures.

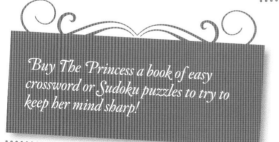

Buy The Princess a book of easy crossword or Sudoku puzzles to try to keep her mind sharp!

Be patient with The Princess and make light of this when possible. But be sure to acknowledge it when she is frustrated.

Don't forget to provide The Princess with a notepad and pen to keep next to her bed. She can jot down "things to do" and also record any messages from doctors or nurses. Buy her an address book to keep next to her bed to have quick access to important numbers, such as doctors, nurses, carpool drivers, and all girlfriends contact numbers. (You can also print up a card with all important phone numbers and pass along to all those involved in The Princess' care. Make several copies for The Princess to keep by all phones throughout her castle.)

PRINCESS' POSSE
(Think about making this index-card size and laminating)

Contact	Home #	Work #	Cellular #	Addr'l #

TREAT HER LIKE
a Princess

*The Princess may find her skin dry during treatment. Palmer's Olive Butter Formula is great for hydrating her skin. She may find her eyes dry, too, so get her some eye lubricant. Check with her doctor first to make sure that is ok.

*Buy The Princess two small fans to keep by her bed and in her bathroom. Hot flashes are a common side effect of chemo!

MOUTH SORES
Buy The Princess baking soda to keep in her bathroom. She can mix it with water and swish the mixture in her mouth when she needs relief.

ACT Fluoride Rinse will provide relief, as well.

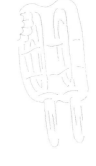

Sorbets, frozen fruits, and popsicles will be welcome treats once the mouth sores set in.

Find out what The Princess' favorite smoothie flavors are and treat her once a week. Some flavors may sting, so check on the developments from time to time!

WEIGHT GAIN

Most people will be surprised to know that many breast cancer patients gain weight. The combination of steroids and the havoc that is wrecked on the hormones contribute to this. The Princess' body may crave certain "comfort" foods. Find out what they are and have them available for her. However, do try and provide healthful alternatives if possible.

For those women who have nausea, make sure that they are replenishing their electrolytes. Keep The Princess well-stocked with saltines and be sure she stays hydrated.

EXERCISE

Encourage The Princess to keep up with her normal regime as much as possible. There is no reason she needs to stop exercising just because she is undergoing treatment. It is extremely important for her mental (as well as physical) health to keep this up. However, make sure The Princess listens to the signals her body is sending her and that she works out accordingly. If she is working out at a gym, buy The Princess some workout gloves that cover her entire hand (like golf or baseball)

TREAT HER LIKE
a Princess

to protect her from the germs that are on the equipment. Depending on her exercise style, have the girlfriends offer to pick her up for a walk or run in the park or for a workout at the gym. Knowing someone is going with her might be all the motivation she needs.

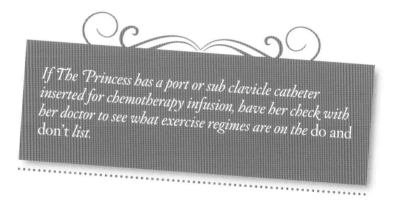

If The Princess has a port or sub clavicle catheter inserted for chemotherapy infusion, have her check with her doctor to see what exercise regimes are on the do and don't list.

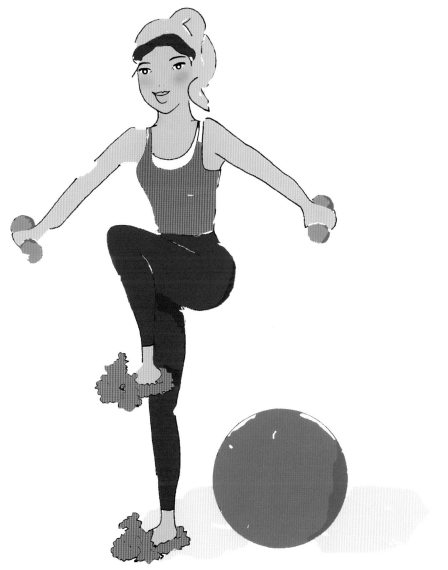

TREAT HER LIKE
a Princess

Chapter 8
SURGERY

The Princess needs to educate herself on all the surgical options available to her.

Many hospitals offer DVDs and pamphlets on surgical choices. A well-informed Princess will have an easier time discussing options with surgeons. Remind The Princess that ultimately she will make the decision regarding the surgery she will have. No one, including the doctors, has the final say but her.

Many volunteers at Breast Clinics are survivors. It is not unusual for the volunteers to offer to "show and tell." Often nicknamed "the flashers," they can provide useful information. Have The Princess ask what surgeries they underwent and when, and to share their experiences. It is helpful to talk to several women.

***

Books and DVDs provide useful information, but they are often very clinical and may provide too much reality for The Princess. Nothing beats seeing a healthy and strong woman who is proud of her new body.

How to Help Your Girlfriend with Breast Cancer

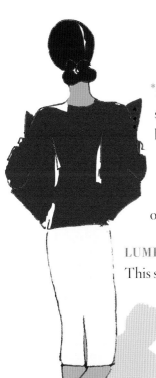

*Suggest The Princess take a picture of her breasts prior to surgery if she is having a bilateral mastectomy. This will be helpful if she is having reconstructive surgery in the future.

SURGICAL OPTIONS

The staging of The Princess' cancer will dictate her surgery options and where it might fall in her treatment plan.

LUMPECTOMY

This surgery involves taking out a portion of the breast tissue. The size of the tumor will determine how much tissue is removed.

A lumpectomy is generally an outpatient procedure. Make sure The Princess has someone to accompany her and bring her home from the hospital.

77

TREAT HER LIKE
a Princess

MASTECTOMY

Mastectomy surgery is the removal of all of the breast tissue. Most patients will also have lymph nodes removed to check for possible cancer.

The Princess may find herself frightened about her sexuality and femininity prior and post surgery.

Before her surgery, gather the girlfriends and throw a "Bra Burning Party." Burn The Princess' bras and then present her with sexy camisoles or nightgowns. How about buying a sheet cake with "boobs" on top. Everyone can take turns being the surgeon!

Unfortunately, most insurance companies only cover a 24-hour stay post mastectomy surgery. Make sure The Princess has received post surgery instructions before she goes home. She will need to get post surgery exercises to help her regain her range of motion. If she is going home with drains, she needs to get specific instructions on how to care for them.

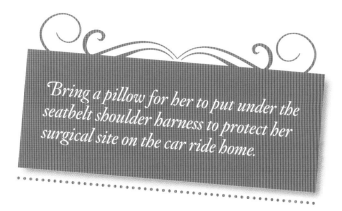

Bring a pillow for her to put under the seatbelt shoulder harness to protect her surgical site on the car ride home.

TREAT HER LIKE
a Princess

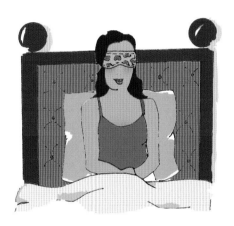

Chapter 9
HOSPITAL CARE

Depending on her surgery, The Princess may require a hospital stay.

There are several things that can be done to make her stay more comfortable.

HOSPITAL CARE PACKAGE

My philosophy is "once a Princess, always a Princess." Make sure The Princess has a care package that includes ear plugs, an eye mask (preferably something in animal print or sequins), lip balm, brush ups, and unscented lotion. (Remember that The Princess might have a heightened sense of smell. Opt for unscented products such as Burt's Bees.)

*Without The Princess' knowledge take pictures of her loved ones (kids, significant others, pets, siblings etc.) prior to her hospital stay. Print the pictures up and scatter them throughout her room.

*Prior to surgery, make sure the Princess has front button down pj's and nightgowns. A pretty bed jacket (think Doris Day!) is perfect to put on over her hospital gown when she has visitors. Also, buy her a brightly colored satin pillowcase to take to the hospital. The Princess can then bring her favorite pillow from home and it will not be confused with the hospital ones!

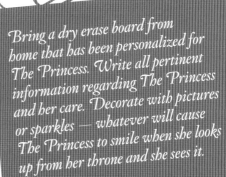

Bring a dry erase board from home that has been personalized for The Princess. Write all pertinent information regarding The Princess and her care. Decorate with pictures or sparkles — whatever will cause The Princess to smile when she looks up from her throne and she sees it.

Small heart-shaped pillows are wonderful post surgery. They fit perfectly under the arm, taking the weight of the arm off the incision site. They also protect from the pressure of the seatbelt. Once home, they make a comfy neck rest!

81

TREAT HER LIKE
a Princess

Leave a large of bowl filled with candy in The Princess' room for the nurses. There's nothing wrong with a little incentive to have the nurses visit The Princess more often!

Antibacterial wipes are refreshing since Princess will be unable to shower. She will also need nonskid slippers and a robe to throw over her shoulders once she is able to get up and walk around.

Make sure she has something to wear home from the hospital that is easy for her to put on. The Princess will not be able to lift her arms. She will need shirts that can fit over her head without using her arms or shirts that button up the front.

HOSPITAL BUDDY
Make sure someone spends the night with The Princess, especially the first night.

The hospital buddy is responsible for telling nurses where to take blood pressure. (In the case that lymph nodes are removed, the arm cuffs should not be used on that arm. If both arms are affected, the cuff will need to be placed on the leg.) One way to ensure that the blood pressure is taken from the correct place is to write in permanent marker "no blood pressure" on the affected arm(s). Have The Princess write this prior to surgery since she may be asleep when the nurses come in. This will be a surefire way to make certain blood pressure is taken correctly.

The nurses will not be able to respond to The Princess' needs as quickly as the hospital buddy, so be prepared. The hospital buddy will need to keep track of The Princess' blood pressure, temperature, medicines, doctor visits and doctor comments.

Prior to surgery, ask The Princess if she has any drug or skin allergies, and keep this information in a notebook. Ask nurses what medications they are giving The Princess and make sure they are not on the "no-no" list. Mistakes can and do happen.

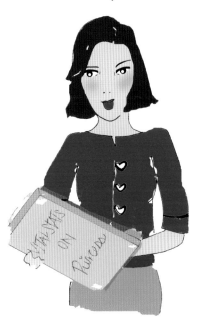

TREAT HER LIKE
a Princess

The most important role of the hospital buddy is that of Police Woman. She will need to monitor phone calls and visitors so that The Princess is not overwhelmed. Make sure this person can sense when

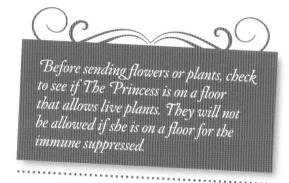

Before sending flowers or plants, check to see if The Princess is on a floor that allows live plants. They will not be allowed if she is on a floor for the immune suppressed.

The Princess is tired. All visits and phone calls should be limited so The Princess can rest. Keep a list of all gifts and flowers The Princess receives. The hospital buddy will also inform the "Webmaster" of all aspects of The Princess' recovery.

HOME SWEET HOME

Once The Princess returns to her palace, make sure she has everything she needs to help her feel comfortable. Fill her prescriptions before she comes home so she will have them when she needs them. Easy-to-serve lunches are helpful. Soups, tuna or chicken salad are nice to have on hand when she has visitors. Make sure her freezer is stocked. This is an especially important time to have the food and activity schedules in order.

Once again, assign a Police Woman to monitor The Princess' phone calls and visitors.

84

HOME CARE PARAPHERNALIA

Some of this depends on The Princess, and some of it depends on the surgery. Make sure she has plenty of pillows to pile around her while she rests. Loose, comfortable clothing (think "lounge wear") is a must—especially pants with draw strings or elastic waists.

If she lives in a two-story house, have The Princess check with her health-care provider to see if they will cover the rental of a hospital bed and walker. These are especially helpful after reconstructive surgery. A potty lift (this can be purchased at most pharmacies) is a lifesaver. Post surgery, The Princess may have limited use of her arms or abs, so the potty lift will be most beneficial!

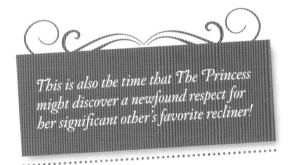

This is also the time that The Princess might discover a newfound respect for her significant other's favorite recliner!

TREAT HER LIKE
a Princess

DRAINS

The Princess will most likely come home with one or two drains post surgery.
If there is a Florence Nightingale girlfriend in the midst, have her assist
The Princess with attention to the drains.

The Princess will be encouraged to do certain exercises to help her regain her
range of motion. However, it is very important for her to take it easy post surgery
in order to ensure a faster recovery. The more active she is, the longer she will
have her drains.

One of the obstacles The Princess will face with her drains (aka canteens) is
how to be fashionable and camouflage them. Before she leaves the hospital,
see if they have a "drain belt" to which she can secure the drains and wear
under her clothing. If not, any soft, cloth belt will do. All The Princess will
need to do is attach the drains to the belt with large safety pins.

Buy The Princess several "Cuddle Duds" camisoles to wear post surgery.
They are soft and will be gentle against her skin as it heals.

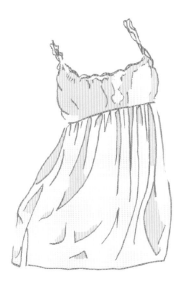

POST SURGERY SENSITIVITY

The reality of mastectomy or lumpectomy surgery may be devastating to The Princess. Think of ways to make her feel feminine and frilly, if that is her style, or sporty, or sharp, or however she has defined herself before the surgery. Help her to love her new healthy body.

Now is the time to get together with the other girlfriends and buy The Princess a gift certificate to Victoria's Secret or Frederick's of Hollywood.

RECONSTRUCTIVE SURGERY

Some breast cancer patients are able to have reconstructive surgery at the time of their mastectomy. However, some may not. Waking up from surgery and finding a void where there once was a breast can be heartbreaking to The Princess. Try making her a CD by downloading songs from iTunes that will inspire her and help her to project the new woman she has become—a Princess who is not only a fighter but one who is strong and beautiful from the inside out.

87

TREAT HER LIKE
a Princess

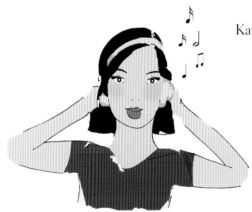

Helen Reddy — *I am Woman, Hear Me Roar*

Gloria Gaynor — *I Will Survive*

Survivor — *Eye of the Tiger*

Wicked Soundtrack — *Defying Gravity*

Bette Midler — *You Gotta Have Friends*

Katrina and the Waves — *I'm Walking on Sunshine*

Pointer Sisters — *Jump*

James Brown — *I Feel Good*

Avril Levine — *Keep Holding On*

Michael Jackson — *Man in the Mirror*

Christina Aguilera — *Beautiful*

Dionne Warwick — *Say a Little Prayer*

George Michael — *Freedom*

Melissa Etheridge — *I Run to You*

Andrew Goldstein — *Thank you for being a Friend*

Carole King — *You've got a Friend*

Smash Mouth — *I get Knocked Down*

Desiree — *You Gotta Be Bold*

Bachman-Turner Overdrive — *You Aint Seen Nothin' Yet*

Beyonce — *Survivor*

Remember not to be judgmental of The Princess. Everyone has their own views regarding their bodies and sexuality. Now is the time to be empathetic.

There are several reconstructive surgery options available for The Princess. Some of these will depend on her treatment plan, her body type, and other issues.

TISSUE OR SKIN-EXPANDERS

This is considered the least involved reconstructive option. It is the most common and has the easiest recovery period. Post mastectomy, The Princess will undergo a surgery where the surgeon inserts an expander beneath the skin and chest muscle (think of a balloon). Over the next several months, liquid is inserted into the expander to gently "stretch" the skin. Once the desired size is achieved, a permanent implant will replace the expander.

TRAMS (TRANSVERSE RECTUS ABDOMINUS MUSCLE) FLAP

This surgery uses extra tissue and muscle from the lower tummy wall. (If The Princess is super model thin, this will most likely not be an option for her!) The surgeon "tunnels" under the skin fat, blood vessels and at least one of the abdominal muscles under the skin to the chest. If there is not enough tissue, some patients opt to have implants. This is a very involved surgery that will require The Princess to be in the hospital for several days. She can expect to be completely out of commission for at least 2 weeks post surgery. She will really need all her support system to be there to pick up the slack! It is very important that she plan ahead and have all her "ducks in a row" prior to surgery! The benefit to this surgery is that The Princess will receive a "tummy tuck" as part of the deal!

FREE FLAP

The Free Flap is very similar to the Trams. However, the blood supply is disconnected and then reconnected in the chest. The surgeon then sews the blood vessels so the blood supply is restored to the tissue. This is a very long and complicated surgery that often requires an overnight stay in ICU to monitor the blood supply. The benefit to this surgery is that the rectus abdominus muscle is not as involved. The recovery is similar to the Trams Flap. The Princess will need 24/7 help for the first two week.

LATISSIMUS DORSI MUSCLE FLAP (BACK TISSUE)

The skin and muscle from The Princess' back are removed and "tunneled" under the skin to the front of the chest to create a pocket. Implants are usually inserted into the pocket.

*If at all possible, once The Princess has healed from her surgery, send a massage therapist to her castle. Find a therapist who can massage her scar tissue and help her regain her range of motion.

THE FINAL FRONTIER!

After the surgery has healed, The Princess will be ready for the final stage of her reconstruction—the making of the nipple.

Many surgeons perform this part of the procedure in their offices. The first part is the construction of the nipple. The surgeon will create the nipple from the new skin. The doctor will have to cut the new breast and stitch the skin in order to form the new nipple. Although, this does not cause The Princess any physical pain, the emotion of having to watch a nipple being created may be too much information for her to absorb. Most doctors will allow The Princess to drive herself. However, check and see if she would like to be chauffeured! She may feel a little woozie after the procedure. Take her out after her appointment to grab a coffee or a see a movie to take her mind off her appointment.

TREAT HER LIKE
a Princess

Once the nipple has healed, the reconstruction surgeon will then tattoo the areola. This is usually done in the office. However, some Princesses opt to go to professional tattoo parlors for a more natural looking nipple. *If The Princess took pictures of her breast(s) prior to surgery have her show the doctor and /or tattoo artist the photos for a visual reference.

*Sassybacks are camisoles with lycra that are comfortable post reconstructive surgery. They provide support and comfort similar to a compression garment but they come in a variety of colors and look better! Make sure to get the ones without underwire support.

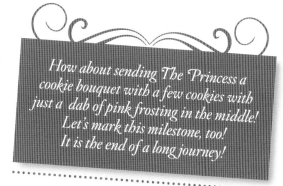

How about sending The Princess a cookie bouquet with a few cookies with just a dab of pink frosting in the middle! Let's mark this milestone, too! It is the end of a long journey!

Prosthesis Shopping

Prior to shopping for prostheses, have The Princess get a prescription from her surgeon. If she had lymph nodes removed, have her get a prescription for a compression garment, too.

Check around the kingdom to see where to be fitted for and purchase prostheses. Many hospitals have shops that sell post mastectomy gear. Check the phone book to see if there are any stores outside of the hospital. She will not be able to be fitted for her permanent prosthesis immediately after surgery, so make sure she has a "trainer" while she is healing. Many of these stores offer options for bathing suits, workout gear, camis, etc. Lands' End offers bathing suits that accommodate prostheses.

Lymphedivas is a company that specializes in decorative compression sleeves. The Princess can even match her compression sleeves with the color of her workout wear. If The Princess has ever longed to be inked, some of their styles offer her a chance to see what she would look like without the permanence of a real tattoo.

The National Lymphedema group offers a website for advice and precautions.

Nordstom's offers a service in which they will take a bra and make a pocket for the prosthesis. All you have to do is ask!

93

TREAT HER LIKE
a Princess

POST MASTECTOMY CARE

Check with The Princess' surgeon for handouts on post mastectomy exercises. The American Cancer Society offers a service called Reach to Recovery that assists patients after mastectomy surgery. If available in her area, they may come to The Princess' castle or the hospital and help her with exercises, give her advice regarding prosthesis choices, compression sleeves and other issues post mastectomy patients face.

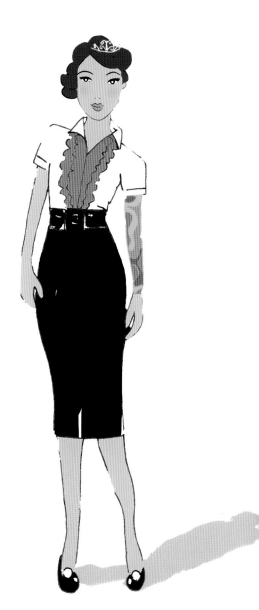

LYMPHEDEMA

Lymphedema is a condition that all breast cancer patients need to be aware of if they have had lymph nodes removed. The Princess will need to be fitted for a compression sleeve that she will need to wear on long car rides, air flights, and when she exercises or does any repetitive movements for any length of time. She will need to ask her surgeon or oncologist for a prescription prior to her fitting.

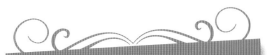

Remind The Princess that the lymphatic drainage system protects us from infection. When that system is compromised, we must protect ourselves! Buy her a festive pair of gardening gloves for all her outdoor digging. Remind her to keep the weightlifting to single digits. Make sure her manicurist is a fanatic about cleanliness. Encourage her to buy her own manicure tools to take with her to each appointment.

***

Lymphedema can rear its ugly head even years after The Princess' surgery. She needs to keep her tiara on forever when it comes to lifting heavy items such as luggage, trash or groceries.

TREAT HER LIKE
a Princess

Cellulitis is a serious problem that all post-mastectomy patients need to be aware of. Cellulitis is a bacterial infection of the skin that enters through a break in the skin. In cancer patients, cellulitis may be caused by lymphedema. *To help The Princess prevent cellulitis remind her to:*

- Avoid using affected arm when receiving vaccines or injections or when having blood drawn.
- Avoid excessive heat—no whirlpools or saunas.
- Always use a hot pad to prevent burns.
- Always use sun screen and wear long sleeves to avoid sun burns.
- Protect skin from cuts and scratches.
- Avoid harsh detergents or deodorants.
- Keep hands and cuticles soft.
- Always bring personal equipment to manicures.

96

MASSAGE THERAPY AND PHYSICAL THERAPY

Both of these therapies can be beneficial to The Princess in helping her regain her range of motion. However, make sure The Princess' therapists are gentle with her arm. There is a huge difference between gently stretching her arm and forcing it. Remind The Princess that she is in control of her body. If a therapist is hurting her or if she feels a "popping" sensation, she must tell them to stop. Overuse or extension of her arm can cause lymphedema.

One therapy in particular that can be beneficial to The Princess is Manual Lymphatic Draining Massage therapy. Have her check in her area to see if there is a licensed therapist.

Regular massages are fine as long as the therapist is told to massage or push up on the affected arm instead of pulling down.

Chapter 10
RADIATION

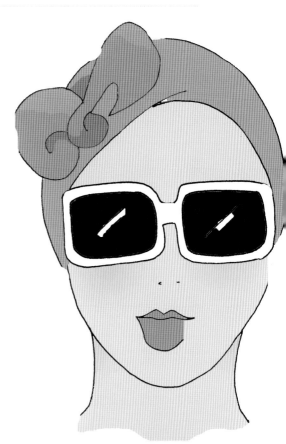

As The Princess begins radiation therapy, the technicians and/or doctors will draw a "map" on her skin in permanent marker. This will remain on her until the completion of her treatment. The markings can rub off on her clothing. Buy her a few nice cotton crewneck T-shirts or turtlenecks to wear during this time. That way, The Princess will not soil her favorite blouse or dress and the cut of the shirt will cover up the markings.

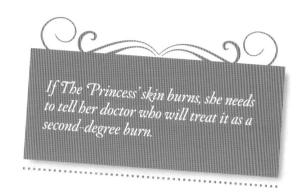

If The Princess' skin burns, she needs to tell her doctor who will treat it as a second-degree burn.

*Some women opt to have their radiation sessions first thing in the morning. This allows them the flexibility to continue on with their activities. Most sessions last only 30 minutes, so if the schedule is not delayed she can be in and out of there in an hour! She will be the darling of the radiation department if she brings a dozen bagels or donuts for the radiology technicians! Often hospital staff is overworked and underappreciated. They will be grateful for the act of kindness.

The Princess will need to ask her doctor what products are allowed during her treatment to protect and heal her skin from burning. Often radiation patients are allowed to use products such as Aqua Phore, Alpha Keri oil, shea and coconut butter.

Chapter 11
CELEBRATE

Take the opportunity to celebrate at every juncture of The Princess' treatment. When she is halfway through treatment—celebrate! When she is finished with chemotherapy—throw a party! If radiation is the last of her treatments, make sure to mark this milestone.

Mark every milestone. When The Princess is halfway through chemo, come to her appointment fully loaded with party hats, blowers, sparkling cider, and plastic champagne flutes! Buy a sheet cake and write a cute quote like "Almost There" or "On the downhill…" Pass the hats, blowers and cake around the unit and get everybody involved! Make it a true celebration! (Leave all the extra goodies with the nurses. They work so hard and deserve a treat too!)

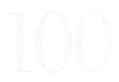

At the end of all her rounds of chemotherapy have a Girlfriend luncheon at someone's home or a favorite quiet restaurant. Have everyone arrive wearing their favorite hat! Have each guest write a note to The Princess saying "Our hats are off to you..." and include an anecdote about her (funny or otherwise)! Take a picture of The Princess with each guest. After the party, make a digital photo album including all the pictures and anecdotes.

If radiation is the last leg of her journey, be sure to have as many girlfriends there as possible for her last treatment. Many hospitals have patients ring a bell at the conclusion of their treatment. If The Princess' hospital does not, start a new tradition. Bring in a dinner bell or office bell and ring in the new healthy year with her in style!

*Find out when The Princess celebrates her anniversary (ironically, it is the day she is diagnosed) and mark this milestone every year!

*Make sure that the Webmaster has access to all pictures taken of The Princess during her treatment. Have her post on the webpage from time to time.

TREAT HER LIKE
a Princess

Acknowledge that this has been a journey filled with highs and lows. The girlfriends and The Princess have all learned a great deal about each other and life. Continue to make opportunities to really appreciate each other. *Now that the journey through cancer treatment is over, don't stop there. Learn to slow down. Make time for each other. Go to lunch. See a movie in the middle of the day. Cherish your friendships.*

POST TREATMENT
You may notice a change in The Princess after the completion of her treatment. While she was in the midst of it, she was most likely in "fighter" mode. Many survivors find that once their treatment is over, they become depressed and anxious of reoccurrence. Be especially sensitive to this and *continue to make your Princess feel regal.*

Be accepting of The Princess' new circle of friends. This does NOT mean that she doesn't love or appreciate you. Please be understanding of their bond and respect her need to be with them. She may not have wanted to join their sorority, but now that she is in it, she is a sister for life.

*If you find The Princess melancholy, suggest that she find local support groups. Many hospitals offer these as well as lecture series and exercise and relaxation classes.

Remember not to fall back into the same fast track and ignore your friendships and speed through life without enjoying one another! Live every day to its fullest!

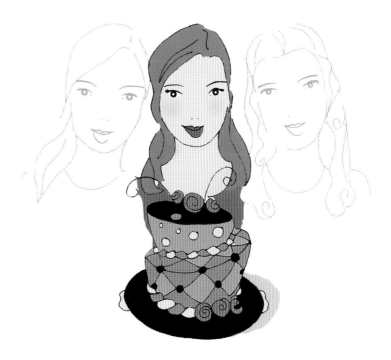

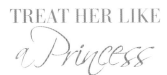
TREAT HER LIKE
a Princess

Chapter 12
I WILL SURVIVE

As The Princess makes the transition from patient to survivor, the girlfriends and The Princess should take a step back and analyze all that they have been through. Stop and realize what a great gift you have all been given. How lucky to be surrounded by so many loving and giving people. Help The Princess to realize what an amazing person she has become. Compliment her on her strength, her perseverance and her faith in beating this beast. Respect how she chooses to live out her life now that she has been transformed into a true "Super Woman." You will find that some Princesses will want to volunteer in the local hospitals, some will join support groups, others will just want to put breast cancer behind them and move on, and others may want to climb the highest mountain and scream, "I am woman, hear me roar!" Any way she goes, just make sure you are there beside her to say, *"we made it!"*

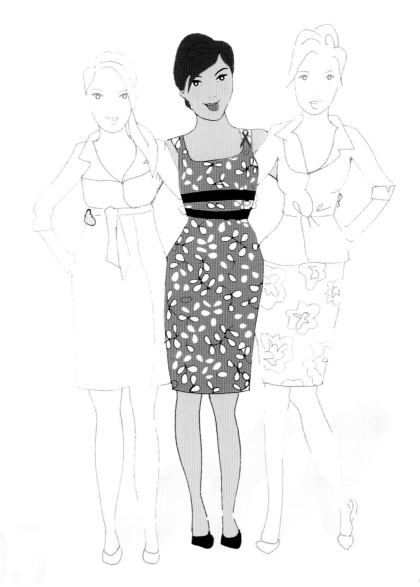

TREAT HER LIKE
a Princess

Royal Court for Princess

_____

_____

Queen Bee(s)

#1 _____

#2 _____

_____

Master of the Meals

#1 _____

#2 _____

_____

Webmaster(s)

#1 _____

#2 _____

_____

Chemo Buddy Scheduler _____

Chemo Buddies

1. _____
2. _____
3. _____
4. _____
5. _____

6. _____
7. _____
8. _____
9. _____
10. _____

Hospital Buddy _____

Kids Organizer _____

Prince Charming's Support Group

1. _____
2. _____

3. _____
4. _____

Castle Control _____

Pet Keeper _____

TREAT HER LIKE
a Princess

SOURCES

www.avoncompany.com — A foundation set up in response to the needs of women and their families to raise funds and awareness for advancing access to care and to finding a cure for breast cancer.

www.beautysociety.com — Offers great and safe products to restore The Princess lush eyelashes.

www.blockbuster.com — Online DVD rentals by mail.

www.burtsbees.com — Great unscented products for chapped and dry skin and lips.

www.cancer.org — For support in your area, visit the "In My Community" section on the website or call 1-800-227-2345 to find a Reach for Recovery volunteer.

www.carecalendar.org — Web-based system to organize meals and other help for families during a time of illness or life-changing event.

www.carepages.com — A community of free websites created by patients and families so they can share information, support and photos.

cindyburnham@comcast.net. Holding it Together Organizer — A helpful patient organizer.

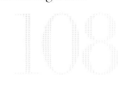

www.cleaningforareason.org—Cleaning services for patients.

Corporate Angel Network—914-328-1313/866-328-1313—Free air transportation for cancer patients traveling to treatment using empty seats on corporate jets.

www.dslrf.org—Mission of the Dr. Susan Love Research Foundation is to eradicate breast cancer and improve the quality of women's health through innovative research, education and advocacy. One million women, one research goal, one revolutionary opportunity - together we can prevent breast cancer.

www.facebook.com—A social networking website that connects people with friends and others.

www.facingourrisk.org—Offers information and support for those women who are genetically at high risk for breast and ovarian cancer.

www.her2support.org—Provides information about the HER2 gene plus message boards.

www.komen.org—Breast cancer information site that offers education and research about causes, treatment, and the search for a cure.

www.landsend.com—Post mastectomy bathing suits.

www.lotsofhelpinghands.com—Website that helps to organize families during their time of need.

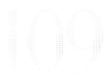

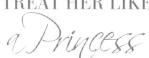

TREAT HER LIKE
a Princess

www.lymphedivas.com—Fashionable compression sleeves.

www.netflix.com—Online DVD rentals by mail.

www.outreachofhope.org—Their mission is to serve suffering people, especially those with cancer and amputation, by offering resources for encouragement, comfort and hope through a personal relationship with Jesus Christ.

www.pinkribbons.org—Using the arts to save lives and improve the quality of life for those touched by breast cancer.

www.planetbuff.com—Offers the entire USA collection of Buff products, including Buff bandanas Buff headgear and Buff wear.

Road to Recovery—800-227-2345—American Cancer Society volunteers provide limited transportation to and from treatment centers.

www.shopbrita.com—Water filtration system and products.

www.thera-wear.com—A great source for inspirational t-shirts and note cards. Thera-wear encourages you to "dress yourself into healthy thinking!"

www.youngsurvival.org—A nonprofit network of breast cancer survivors and supporters dedicated to the concerns and issues unique to young women and breast cancer.

GLOSSARY

Here is a little more explanation of some terms used in this book:

Breast Cancer—Uncontrolled growth of abnormal breast cells.

BRCa1 (Breast Cancer 1, Early onset)—A human gene in which some mutations are associated with significant increase in the risk of breast cancer and other cancers.

BRCa2 (Breast Cancer 2, Type 2 susceptibility protein)—Certain variations of this gene cause an increased risk for breast cancer and other cancers.

Breast Prosthesis—Artificial breast form that can be worn under clothing post mastectomy.

Cellulitis—A bacterial infection of the skin that enters through breaks in the skin. Lymphedema may cause this in cancer patients.

Chemotherapy—Treatment with drugs to destroy cancer cells.

Estrogen Receptor Tumors—Tumors that are sensitive to estrogen hormones.

Free Flap—Reconstructive surgery option similar to the TRAMs with the exception that the blood supply is disconnected and then reconnected in the chest. The blood vessels are sewn to restore blood supply to the tissue. Implants are sometimes used to achieve desired size.

TREAT HER LIKE
a Princess

HER/neu—(Human epidermal growth factor receptor 2) This protein is involved in the growth of some cancer cells.

Inflammatory Breast Cancer—Special class of cancer where the breast looks inflamed or infected because of its red appearance and feels warm to the touch. The skin shows signs of ridges or may have a pitted appearance.

Latisimus—Reconstructive surgery option where the skin and muscle from the back are removed and "tunneled" under the skin to the front of the chest to create a pocket. Implants are usually inserted into the pocket to achieve the desired size.

Lumpectomy—Surgery to remove lump along with a small margin of normal breast tissue around it.

Lymphatic Drainage System—Moves protein and fluid from the body tissues back into the bloodstream. Also acts as a filter removing malignant and bacterial cells out of the bloodstream.

Lymphedema—Swelling of the arm caused by the excess of fluid. May occur after lymph nodes are removed or following radiation. It can be temporary or permanent. It can happen immediately or any time later.

Lymph nodes—Glands found throughout the body that help defend against foreign invaders such as bacteria.

Malignant—Cancerous.

Mastectomy—Surgical removal of the breast and some surrounding tissue.

Novaldex/Tamoxifen—Estrogen blocker used in treating breast cancer.

Primary Tumor—The original tumor.

Raloxifene/Evista—Selective Estrogen Receptor Modulators (SERMs) Synthetic drug that blocks the action of estrogen.

Sentinel Node Biopsy—Diagnostic procedure used to determine whether breast cancer has spread to auxiliary lymph nodes (i.e.—lymph nodes under the arm.)

Staging—Tests and exams done before any kind of definitive treatment to determine if cancer has spread.

Tissue Expander—Reconstructive surgery option where an expander is inserted beneath the skin and chest muscle. Over time, liquid is slowly inserted into the expander(s) to gently "stretch" the skin. A permanent implant replaces the expander once the desired size is achieved.

Trams Flap—Reconstructive surgery option where the surgeon "tunnels" skin, fat, blood vessels and at least one of the abdominal muscles under the skin to the chest to create the new breast(s). Some patients opt for implants to achieve desired size.

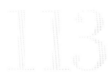

ACKNOWLEDGEMENTS

To my amazing Big Fat Greek Family: Thank you for always being there for me, for supporting me in all my endeavors, for lifting me up when I was down and, above all, for loving me for me:

Mom, you are my sunshine! Thank you for teaching me to always look on the bright side.

Vicki, thank you for dedicating yourself to me and my family for 2 years. You are an inspiration for your unselfishness and unwavering love.

Peter and Thad, thank you for always making me feel like a Princess.

Sarah and Helene, thank you for truly being my sisters in every sense of the word.

Thea Mary, thank you for being my inspiration and role model. I pray that one day I too can claim to be a 50-year survivor.

Uncle Jim, my birthday twin, thank you for being my surrogate father whom I adore.

The Hazen Clan, thank you for your support from both near and far. Barbara, we are not only daughter- and mother-in-law, but now also sisters in the journey.

Aunt Katherine and Uncle Nick, thank you for guiding and supporting me.

Dianna, Peter, Ted and Bryan, and Demetri, Thane, Caitlin, Elizabeth, Claire, John, Thomas, James, Isabella, CeCe, Mary and John, thank you for your unending love.

To the memory of my amazing father: thank you for always being a "best friend" to one and all.

To my amazing Girlfriends: the true inspiration for this book. Without you, *Treat Her Like a Princess* would not have happened. I am so blessed to be surrounded by the most amazing group of women. I will forever be indebted to you all.

Kris, my pethera. You always made sure there was a meal on the table and I was resting.

Ellen, you made sure no one interfered with our running time.

The AOS gals, you picked up the slack and made me smile.

Book Club, you created the "Scarf Party."

Pucci Minkies, who could ask for anything more than Galveston and durags?

TREAT HER LIKE
a Princess

Greek Girls, I loved resurrecting Girls Night. When is the next one? Frosty is lonely!

My extended Greek family, you were always there with a home-cooked meal.

Fr. George, you provided spiritual guidance and emotional support.

Ila, you truly have healing hands and a heart of gold.

Shelley, always smiling and making me laugh.

Drs. Rivera, Ames, Bucholtz, Baldwin, and Beevers, you are the most awesome and brilliant team of doctors.

All the nurses at M.D. Anderson. Thank you for taking care of me and restoring my health.

Lucy and Ellen, my incredible publishers and their team at Bright Sky Press, thank you for believing in me and in The Princess.

Jennifer, my talented illustrator, I have much admiration for the way you have brought the Princess and her girlfriends to life.

And, *to all of you* who sent e-mails, letters, gifts and love throughout my treatment, I am forever grateful.

ABOUT THE AUTHOR

Sassy, determined and unstoppably positive, Denise Dameris Hazen met Stage 3 cancer with the kind of vigor and fortitude that could put a combat marine to shame. Throughout her treatment, Denise allowed herself to be filmed by a CNN film crew for the documentary *Taming the Beast*. As she faced seventeen rounds of chemotherapy, a double mastectomy and six weeks of daily radiation, Denise sent a clear message to other women: Not only is it possible to endure breast cancer treatment, but you can emerge on the other side even stronger than before. Now, in *Treat Her Like a Princess* she details the thoughtful and loving ways that her friends supported her through her battle.

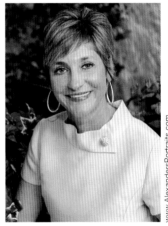

www.AlexandersPortraits.com

Denise lives in Houston, Texas, with her husband, Charles, and their children, Catherine and Nicholas. She continues to offer personal support, insight and love to women diagnosed with breast cancer as well as volunteering with Pink Ribbons Project: In Motion Against Breast Cancer.

TREAT HER LIKE
a Princess

ABOUT THE ILLUSTRATOR

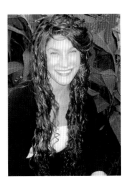

Jennifer Procell studies at The Art Institute of Houston and enoys illustrating and computer-generated imagery. Through her mother, who routinely works with breast cancer survivors, Jennifer met Denise and quickly came to hold her and her family in the highest regard. When Jennifer learned of the concept for the book, she was thrilled at the opportunity to use her artistic skills to promote such an uplifting and meaningful message.

JOURNAL

TREAT HER LIKE
a Princess

....

....

....

....

....

....

....

....

....

....

....

120

TREAT HER LIKE
a Princess

TREAT HER LIKE
a Princess

TREAT HER LIKE
a Princess

127

TREAT HER LIKE
a Princess

Appomattox Regional Library System
Hopewell, Virginia 23860
05/13